Essential Oils for Healing

Disclaimer

Summary

Essential oils are derived from plants and flower. Many medical benefits can be obtained from essential oils, these oils can also help you recover from infections, burns, swelling, arthritis and more. This book will open your eyes to the wonders that essential oils bestow. This book covers the following topics:

- What are essential oils and how are they beneficial?

- The prominence of essential oils in the history of different countries

- Common facts about essential oils

- How essential oil is distilled from plants and flowers.

- The 9 types of essential oils, their benefits, application procedures and precautions

- How safe are essentials to use?

- Factors to be aware of when using these oils

- Emergency procedures

- How to properly test them on your skin

Contents

Introduction to Essential Oils

Do you know that essential oils are a plant's knight in shining armor? Their beautiful and sweet-smelling aroma is just a guise to hide their powerful medicinal powers. Essential oils do not only act as a plant's savior by protecting them from insects, bad weather and disease, but they also help humans in several ways. Their medicinal properties contain antiseptic, anti-allergic, antiviral, and anesthetic and various other properties that help you stay strong and look good. Have you ever wondered why nature such as flowers and plants smell so nice? This is nature's way to beckon and lure you to take a whiff. One sniff of the scent can send you into another world. However, the scent that emanates from flowers and plants is truly incomparable to the synthetic versions of essential oils you find in fragrances. Nevertheless, this was not the real intention of nature's sweet smelling gift.

The intention of essential oils is to help your inner and outer self-thrive. Essential oils are a nature's way of giving back to you. The lists of benefits they include are so numerous that it can take all day to explain the individual advantages of all the essential oils.

They can be combined to create magical healing potions that will help reduce ailments such as rashes, fever, allergies and more. Moreover, if you are struggling with weight loss or worried about your physical appearance, essential oils can also help you achieve flawless skin and a slim waist.

So, why go for over the counter drugs? You can use nature's gift of essential oils to keep you glowing.

The Historical Roots of Essential Oils

The cavemen were the first human beings to discover the healing properties of essential oils. However, this is not the only time in history that people have used essential oils for medical purposes. Before modern medicine was discovered, the Egyptians, Chinese, Indians, Greeks, Persians, Europeans and Romans all used the oils to heal the sick.

A closer inspection of each country's history reveals the significance of essential oils. Then, in 1907, European doctors revived the concept of essential oils in the form of aromatherapy. The following list below details the usage of essential oils in each country's history.

Egypt
The Egyptians are known as the architects of medicine. Their expertise in medicine is still regarded as a major contribution to the medical field. The Egyptians, during 4500 B.C.E., learned about the medical benefits of essential oils. They took the extracted oil from the plants and flowers such as grapes, cumin, aniseed, cedar, castor oil, coriander, garlic, and watermelon and converted it into powders or pills. However, only the Egyptian Pharaohs and Priests were permitted to use these aromatic oils.

China
Between 2697 – 2597 B.C.E., Huang Ti, the emperor of China at the time, discovered essential oils during his reign. The Emperor developed ways to use essentials oils as medicine. Later on, the Emperor went on to create a book centered on the many uses of essential oil. Even today, doctors practicing eastern medicine value his book.

India

Ayurveda is the practice of using essential oils to treat various diseases, which originated in India almost 3000 years ago. The concept was captured in various books that were written in Sanskrit and the use of Ayurveda treatment became widely popularized during the Bubonic Plague, which hit India, as essential oils of different kinds were used to treat the infected people.

Greece

The Greeks were exposed to essential oils when the Greek soldiers traveled to India. The exposure to aromatic oils led Hypocrites, a Greek doctor, to research the plants and flowers producing the oil. Hypocrites went on to examine more than 300 plants, which included peppermint, cumin and thyme. The doctor is referred to as the Father of Medicine in Greek history.

Rome

The Roman doctors discovered essential oils during the fall of the Roman Empire. They collected books written by Greek doctors Hypocrites and Galen when they fled. Both Galen and Hypocrites were accomplished medical researchers mastering in philosophy, surgery, and philosophy during the Greek Empire. The books were then translated into several languages such as Arabic and Persian.

Persia

In Persia, a child prodigy was born by the name of Ali-Ibn-Sana. At the age of 12, Ali-Ibn-Sana wrote about the effects of 800 plants on the human body. Historians credit this child prodigy as inventing the methods of distilling essential oils.

Europe

René-Maurice Gattefossé of France was a chemist who investigated the medical properties of essential oils and how they can be used to cure certain illnesses. Nicholas Culpeper was an English botanist, herbalist, physician, and astrologer who were credited with compiling a book of essential oil remedies.

Facts about Essential Oils

You already know that essential oils are a prominent part of the fabric of medicinal history in many countries. In recent times, the wonderful healing properties of these oils have not gone unnoticed. In the modern age, people began using essential oils to fight off various illnesses. This exposed people to a new kind of therapeutic therapy known as aromatherapy.

Aromatherapy took advantage of the following therapeutic properties of essential oils:

1. **Bacteriostatic** - stops the growth of bacteria.

2. **Lipophilic** - penetrates through the skin and into the internal organs.

3. **Bactericide** - destroys existing bacteria from body.

4. **Cytophylactic** - aids in the renewal of cells.

5. **Antiseptic** - fights off infections from body such as cuts, burns and bruises.

6. **Adaptogens** - have a quick and flexible response time.

Most people are now seeking alternative and natural treatments to heal their ailments. Those people who want to seek alternative treatments have realized the negative side effects of modern drugs. However, some people are still dependent on current drugs and over-the-counter medicines. However, the paradigm of taking pills is gradually shifting as more and more people are trying alternate ways to heal themselves.

Essential Oils: The Creation

There is more to essential oils than just smelling wonderful. Their soothing scent when inhaled ingested or put on one's body can trigger the body's healing process. These little drops of liquid are distilled from fruit, flowers, seeds, plants, roots, leaves, and barks. The process of distilling essential oil is a meticulous process where the person needs to acquire about three million of plants and flowers to yield a pound of essential oil. Depending on the type of flower or plant, the number of flowers and plants needed to yield a pound of essential oil.

Distillation Process

The three types of distillation processes are water distillation, water and steam distillation and steam distillation. In order to conduct a distillation process, you need to place a plant or flower inside the still and seal it. Then the water or steam will slowly break the material inside, thus removing the unstable components of the plant. The components will then will rise and go into the condenser. When the condenser cools the liquid down, they turn into oil.

Essential Oils: The Magical Cure

If you need healing, then essential oils can do the trick. There are over a hundred essential oils found in the world. Most importantly, when combined they have unlimited number of uses. Some of the illnesses that essential oils can cure are:

1. Arthritis

2. Allergies

3. Asthma

4. Wounds and Cuts

5. Indigestion

6. Swelling

7. Headaches

8. Anxiety, fatigue and stress

9. Nausea

10. Insomnia

In addition to healing illness associated with the body, they also work miraculously for healing skin conditions such as wrinkles, dry skin, eczema, sunburn, scabies, fungal infections, rashes, scarring and much more. These miracle oils will help you stay healthy not just from the inside, but on the outside as well.

Types of Essential Oils

When the Egyptians discovered essential oils 6,000 years ago, they kept their discovery hidden, as if it was gold, going so far as to ban the Egyptian people from using it. It was only available to the rulers of the kingdom. However, now, essential oils are found on store shelves, at the doctor's, with medical herbalists and sometimes even in your food. Why was that, suddenly, essential oils were all over the place? It was because they contained precious therapeutic substances that could heal people in magnificent ways. Moreover, they are natural and pure.

Basil Essential Oil

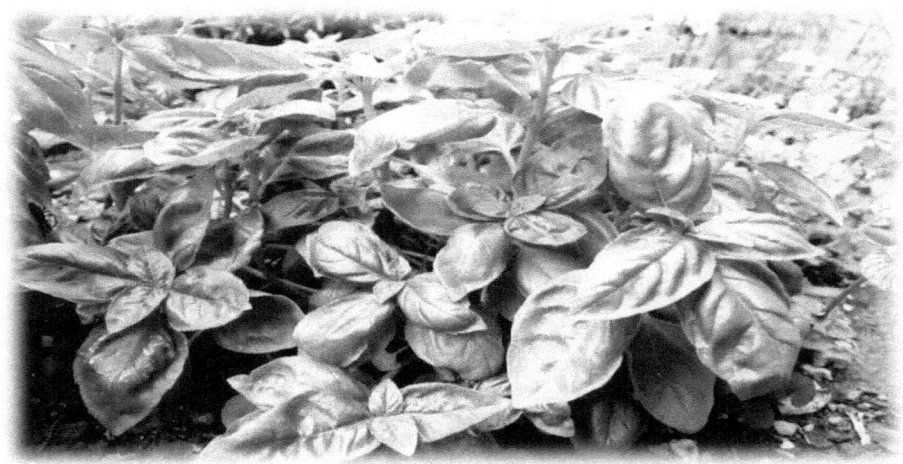

Healing Powers of Basil Essential Oil

You might have come across basil when eating Italian or Mediterranean food. You probably would have put them aside as you are not a goat and don't prefer the taste of leaves in your mouth. You may change your stance on consuming basil, however, after you hear about the numerous benefits it offers.

Basil's healing properties are found in its seeds and leaves, which contain anti-inflammatory, antiviral, anti-infectious, disinfectant, decongestant and antibacterial properties. For this reason, basil has a huge fan base in India, Southeast Asia, Central Asia and Europe as they consistently make it a part of their diet and cuisines.

The Health Benefits of Basil Essential Oil

1. By putting basil oil on your skin and hair, your skin will brighten, your face will look fresh, and your hair will become bouncy and soft. Basil oil can also reduce the appearance of skin diseases.

2. If your stomach is giving you problems and you suffer from digestive ailments such as constipation, indigestion, flatulence and stomach cramps, then basil oil can help loosen up your digestive system giving you quick relief.

3. Basil oil is also quick at relieving you from illnesses such as the flu, the common cold, whooping cough, and fever.

4. If you suffer from bronchitis, asthma, coughs and allergies, basil oil is a good solution for illnesses associated with the respiratory system.

5. Due to Basil oil's antibacterial properties, it can become useful in disinfecting and healing wounds, skin infections, bladder infections and viral infections.

6. Basil oil can help in reducing stress, mental fatigue, migraines, nervous tensions and depression.

7. Basil oil is also an effective pain reliever for treating ailments such as bruises, sprains, wounds, burns and other minor injuries.

8. Ingesting basil oil can improve the flow of blood and the metabolic functions. You can put a drop of it in your food as well.

9. Basil oil is also useful in treating bloodshot eyes and eyestrain.

10. If you feel nauseous, then you can use basil oil as a quick and effective remedy.

11. For itchy stings and bites, basil oil can reduce the urge to scratch them.

Applying Basil Essential Oil

1. **Internal Application**- Although ingesting basil oil is not advised, you can consume basil oil after diluting it in water, honey or when cooking.

2. **Topical Application**- You can apply basil oil directly to your skin or mix it with another essential oil and then apply it to the skin.

3. **Aromatic Application**- You can inhale the fumes through a candle or breathe them in directly.

Basil Essential Oil: Precautions

a) For persons above the age of six, always dilute basil oil before ingesting or applying it.

b) Most importantly, use of basil oil should be avoided during pregnancy or when breastfeeding. Instead, you can use fresh basil leaves and add them to your dinner.

c) A person with epilepsy should avoid using this oil as the smell of the oil may trigger seizures.

d) People with sensitive skin should always test the oil on a part of their skin first.

Clove Essential Oil

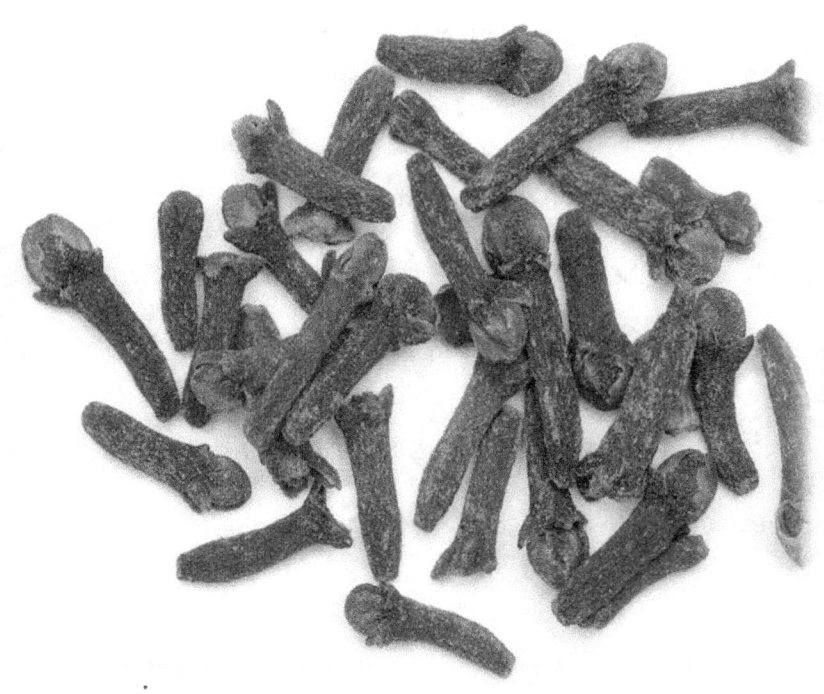

Healing Powers of Clove Essential Oil

If you have a toothpaste or mouthwash at home, look at the ingredient list; you will discover that clove is a primary ingredient. The medicinal properties of clove are located in its flower bud, which contains antifungal, antiviral, antimicrobial, antiseptic, and aphrodisiac benefits. Cloves are also a main ingredient in several Chinese and Indian recipes. You can incorporate cloves in food in either solid, powder, or oil form. By incorporating cloves into your diet, you can receive many health benefits.

The Health Benefits of Clove Essential Oil

1. The antiseptic properties of cloves can be used to apply to cuts, wounds, scabies, fungal infections, bee stings and insect bites, bruises and other minor injuries.

2. Since clove essential oil is an active ingredient in many oral care products, if you ever have a toothache, you can put a drop of oil on the cavity. Also, you can use clove oil for mouth ulcers and sore gums. Furthermore, people with sore throats use clove oil to gargle and remove bad breath.

3. Babies can also benefit from using clove oil. On a teething baby, you can put clove oil onto their gums to ease their discomfort and pain. Since clove oil is very strong, you should dilute before putting it on the baby's gums.

4. Clove oil is a natural remedy to treat acne, diminish wrinkles, and increase blood circulation. You should never put clove oil directly onto your skin, instead put a few drops of oil onto a dry cloth.

5. If you are feeling tired or stressed, use clove oil to stimulate your mind and body. Clove oil works by reducing exhaustion and fatigue. You will be left feeling fresh and free.

6. Insomniacs can use clove oil as a sleeping aid.

7. Clove essential oils can help neural disorder sufferers going through depression, anxiety, and in some cases with memory loss.

8. Headaches, swelling, and muscle pains are also curable with clove oil. You can apply a small amount of clove oil at the base of your neck, which is the culprit of causing headaches and migraines. For reducing muscle pain, just apply directly to the area.

9. To unclog blocked nasal passages, inhale the fumes produced by cloves.

10. An earache can be reduced by combining warm clove oil and sesame oil and putting a few drops of the mixture into the ear.

11. For hiccups, nausea, gas and other indigestion problems, use clove oil. It can also help reduce morning sickness. If you can't ingest it due to its very bitter and strong taste, then you can apply it on a pillow, this way you can inhale the smell of clove oil while you sleep.

12. By ingesting clove oil, your metabolism gets a boost by increasing the flow of blood and decreasing the temperature of the body. In addition, the occurrence of symptoms associated with diabetes such as death, amputations and other complications can be reduced.

13. Clove is a blood-purifying essential oil. You can cleanse your blood by inhaling the odor of clove oil, which, in return, gives your immune system a much needed boost.

Applying Clove Essential Oil

1. **Internal Application** - You can consume clove oil by putting a few drops of oil in food when cooking.

2. **Topical Application** - You can apply clove oil directly on to your skin or on the part of the body that's in pain.

3. **Aromatic Application** - You can inhale clove oil by diluting the clove oil in water and letting it boil on the stove, thus filling the room with the aroma of clove essential oil.

4. **Dilute Application** - Clove is a very strong essential oil that shouldn't be consumed alone. So, when you use clove oil as treatment, remember to dilute it beforehand. Even when applied on to the skin, it needs to be diluted with another essential oil.

Clove Essential Oils: Precautions

a) It is pertinent to understand that diluting the clove oil before application and consumption is extremely necessary. If you do not dilute it, then you risk of getting allergic reactions—especially people with sensitive skin.

b) When putting the clove on your teeth or gums, you should cautiously apply it to sides of your mouth. If applied in haste, then it can burn your mouth. Also, don't leave the clove oil in the mouth for long, instead gargle with water after a few minutes.

c) Don't apply clove essential oil to your skin, insides of the mouth and gums on a regular basis, but give gaps between days.

d) You should try not to inhale the vapors that emanate from clove cigarettes as it can cause restricted breathing and lung diseases. If you do wish to inhale, then put a few drops of oil on a piece of fabric, bring towards your nose to inhale the aroma.

e) Again, when giving clove oil to infants to relieve toothaches, remember to dilute the oil profusely with a different oil or water.

f) Pregnant and breastfeeding women should avoid clove oil. If it must be used, it should be taken in small doses.

g) People with bleeding disorders should avoid taking clove oil as it contains a chemical called eugenol, which slows down blood clotting. In addition, you should stop using clove oil for two weeks prior to surgery to prevent from bleeding too much during or after the operation.

Cypress Essential Oil

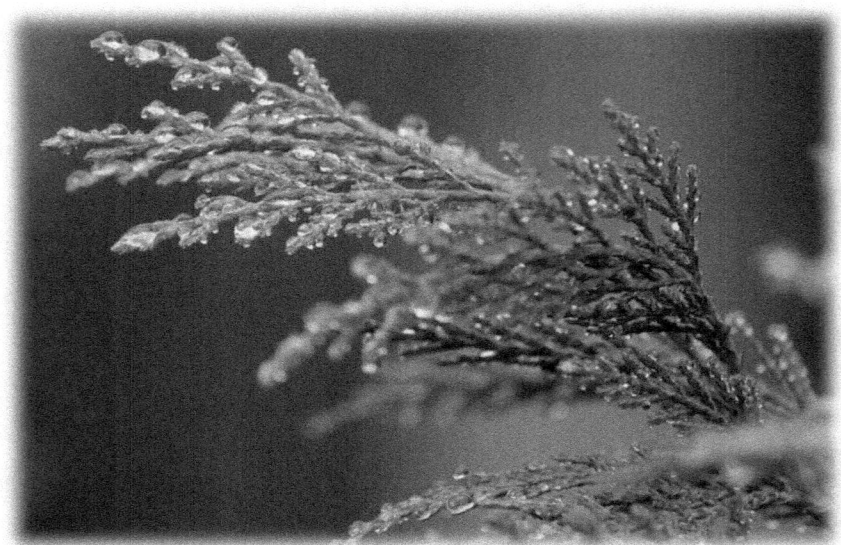

Healing Powers of Cypress Essential Oil

What's ironic about cypress trees is that centuries ago the Romans and the Greeks planted cypress trees around graveyards and burial grounds, but at the same time extracted essential oil from them to treat various conditions. Still today, cypress essential oil's importance is relevant amongst people who prefer to treat illnesses with natural remedies.

Cypress essential oil can be used to treat chronic pain, the flu, strokes, tuberculosis and more. These ancient sources of nutrition and medicine contain antiseptic, diuretic, hepatic, and astringent properties. In addition, they are also used as a sedative and respiratory tonic. These beneficial properties are extracted from the twigs, needles, and stems through the steam distilling process.

The Health Benefits of Cypress Essential Oil

1. Cypress essential oil helps to tighten skin around the muscles, body, and face, prevents hair from becoming greasy and strengthens gums and teeth.

2. Instead of using creams and lotions, use cypress oil to treat internal and external cuts and wounds.

3. One thing that cypress oil is really good for is reducing the rate of spasms. Spasms can occur in the intestines, the limbs, and the respiratory system. Apart from reducing spasms, it also helps to alleviate convulsions, cramps, spasmodic cholera and muscle pulls.

4. It's said that the more you urinate, the more weight you will lose. Consuming drops of cypress essential oil will do just that. It will increase urination and eliminate waste and fat out of the body. Moreover, it increases metabolism, eliminates gas and stops it from developing in the intestines. Also, it eliminates excess water and decreases swelling.

5. Most importantly, people with blood pressure problems can take cypress oil to reduce their blood pressure. Cypress oil can also help remove toxins from the body, as well as cleansing out the kidneys.

6. Cypress essential oil is often deemed as live-saving oil as it contains a medical property called hemostatic. For instance, if a person is losing blood rather quickly, cypress oil can speed up the blood clotting process.

7. Taking cypress essential oil during illnesses that clog up lungs can help eliminate and reduce phlegm build up. It also reduces congestion and coughs, thus making cypress oil a good remedy for sicknesses such as the flu or a runny nose.

8. Skin-related problems like acne can become a nightmare for some people. Therefore, when creams don't work, people should lean towards treating their face with nature-made cypress essential oil. The oil keeps dirt from clogging up the skin's pores and increases sweating. In fact, increased sweating helps cleanse the body of toxins, which help in keeping your skin clean.

9. The liver can benefit from the healing advantages of cypress oil. The oil works as a defender for the liver as it releases the bile from it as well as prevents diseases and common infections from finding their way into the liver.

10. Overanxious people suffering from anxiety and stress can take the oil as a sedative to relax the mind and body. This oil is beneficial for people who are going through trauma, shock, or severe depression.

Applying Cypress Essential Oil

1. **Topical Application** - You can apply cypress oil directly on to your skin or the part of the body that's in pain.

2. **Aromatic Application** - Cypress essential oil has a very strong smell that you can use as a deodorant. You can even add the oil to your footbath to eliminate bacteria that make your feet smell bad. You can also spray it in your house to eliminate foul odor. Plus, breathing the odor will help clear out your lungs.

3. **Neat Application** - This oil doesn't require dilution and can be applied directly to the skin, but before applying do apply a small amount on your skin to determine if the oil suits your skin type or not.

Cypress Essential Oil: Precautions

a) People with hypertension should avoid using this oil.

b) Pregnant women should avoid taking this oil during pregnancy.

c) If you are recovering from a surgery, you should ask your doctor before using cypress oil.

Lavender Essential Oil

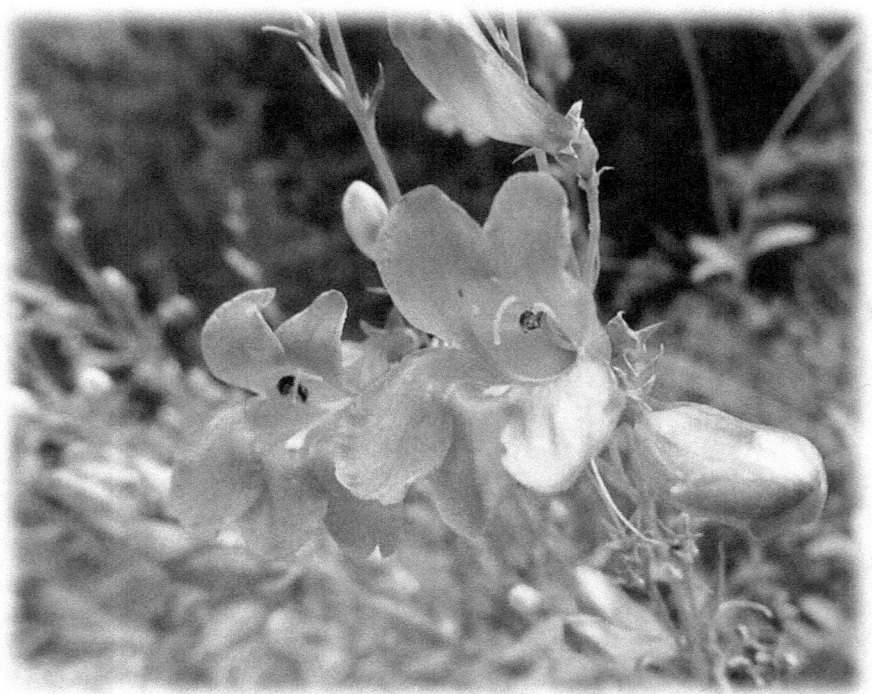

Healing Powers of Lavender Essential Oil

Ever wonder from where potpourri gets its distinct smell from? Its scent is actually derived from dried plants and flowers. Lavender is one type of flower that is often used to make potpourri. The smell of lavender oil is sweet and pleasant. People use the lavender flowers to scent their houses, rooms, closets and bathrooms, but there is more to lavender flowers than just their smell. They have many medical purposes such as antiseptic, antifungal, anti-infectious, and anti-inflammatory properties.

These properties serve a vital purpose in reducing conditions such as blisters, boils, burns, insect bites, cold sores, gangrene, chicken pox, insomnia, mood swings, pains and many more conditions. Lavender comes in various forms including gels, lotions, oils and soaps.

The Health Benefits of Lavender Essential Oil

1. During bug season, a bottle of lavender essential oil helps to ward off flies. With lavender oil applied on your arms and legs, you can go outside with ease, and you can even put the oil on bitten areas of your body. Due to lavender oil's bug repellent properties, it is the main ingredient found in many bug repellent sprays.

2. Having trouble sleeping? If you are not getting enough hours of sleep each day, try scenting your pillow, bed, or room with lavender essential oil.

3. This oil has exhibited great qualities for combating depression, anxiety, headaches, and migraines. Also, if you feel jumpy on certain days and need to calm down your nerves, try inhaling the smell of lavender oil. You can dab the oil on a handkerchief and inhale deeply.

4. If you are prone to getting red inflamed bumps on your face, then the use of lavender scented lotion, soap or oil will help protect your skin from skin diseases like acne. Additionally, regular use of lavender oil prevents and reduces irritation, scarring and infection from occurring in the future.

5. Lavender essential oil is an excellent substitute for ice packs and pain meds. So if you are having muscular pains, sore muscles, sprains, rheumatism, joint pains and backaches, you should massage your body with lavender oil. It will alleviate the pain.

6. Urinary infections can be painful and affect urine build up. Lavender oil can be used to reduce inflammation, cystitis, and cramps associated with urinary infections.

7. Use lavender essential oil to relieve yourself of symptoms of bronchitis, flu, tonsillitis, cough, whooping cough, sinus congestion, phlegm and laryngitis.

8. Lavender oil works well on treating infested hair. All you have to do is to massage the scalp to get rid of unwanted nits, eggs, and lice. Men and women can also use lavender oil to reduce baldness by inducing hair growth.

9. It can increase the flow of blood, decrease blood pressure, boost health, and build muscle strength. This means that the increased blood flow helps to circulate the blood in your body, and in return keeps your skin feeling healthy and fresh.

10. Lavender oil helps your digestion system function better. The oil is also advantageous in fueling the making of bile and gastric juices. In doing so, it's helping to move food around in the intestines and treating such ailments as gas, indigestion, vomiting, colic, diarrhea and stomach pain

11. This oil functions as an antiviral and antibacterial medicine. These two traits found in the lavender oil works well to eliminate rare diseases. Rare diseases like typhoid, tuberculosis and diphtheria.

12. Apart from treating acne, lavender oil also reduces the signs of aging, wounds, burns, psoriasis, cuts and sunburns.

Applying Lavender Essential Oil

1. **Topical Application** - You can apply lavender on your skin without diluting it with another essential oil. You can apply before going out, apply it as a sunscreen, and use it as massage oil.

2. **Aromatic Application** - Lavender essential oils have numerous aromatic uses. You can dab it onto your pillow, spray it around your room or car, or light lavender scented candles around your house.

Lavender Essential Oil: Precautions

a) A woman who is either expecting or breastfeeding should not smell or even put lavender oil on her skin.

b) Diabetic patients should also avoid coming in close contact with lavender oil.

c) People with sensitive skin should avoid applying it to their skin as it can result in allergic reactions. However, they can test the oil against their skin to determine if an allergic reaction occurs or not.

d) Excessive use of lavender oil overtime can cause headaches, vomiting and nausea.

e) Never, ever, consume lavender oil as it can cause serious and dangerous side effects. Consuming lavender oil causes a person's vision to get blurry, restricts breathing, can cause vomiting, upset stomach and burning eyes. However, you can inhale lavender oil.

Cinnamon Essential Oil

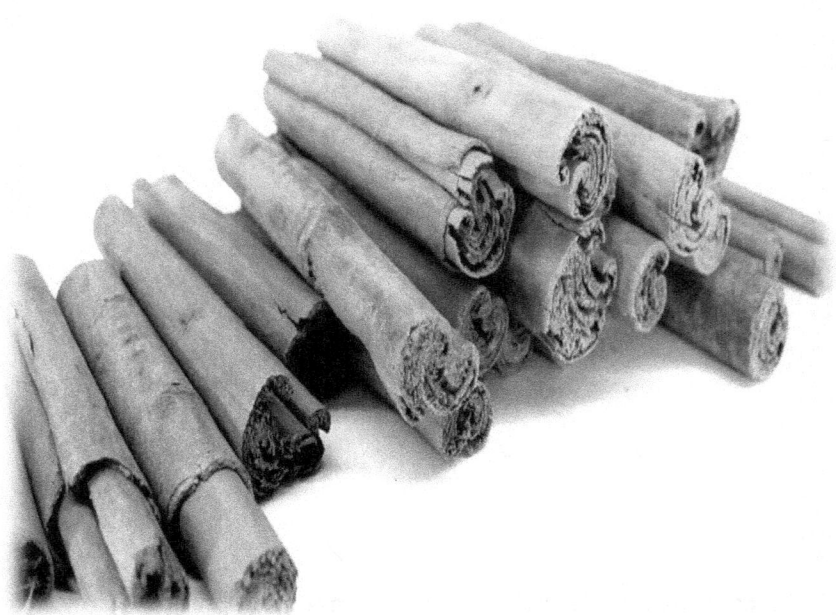

Healing Powers of Cinnamon Essential Oil

The most common use of cinnamon is in cooking food. Its presence in food enhances the dish's taste. In addition to being used for flavoring, cinnamon can also be used as medicine. Knowing the benefits of cinnamon, people began to develop an alternate version of cinnamon—cinnamon essential oil.

A culture that found the use of cinnamon essential to be beneficial was India. India's famous and historical medical system called Ayurveda recognized the medicinal properties of cinnamon and incorporated it into their traditional medical treatments.

Now, cinnamon-distilled-into-cinnamon essential oil is famously used as a form of treatment for colds, digestive problems, yeast infections, arthritis and diarrhea. Cinnamon essential oil has astringent, antibacterial, antimicrobial and anti-clotting properties. Its medical properties are found in its bark, which is used to make pure and natural cinnamon oil.

The Health Benefits of Cinnamon Essential Oil

1. The aroma of cinnamon oil increases brain activity. People suffering from the loss of memory or anxiety should inhale the scent of cinnamon oil at least once a day. Although there is no harm, they can inhale the cinnamon oil more than once in a day. Furthermore, breathing in cinnamon oil leads to an increase in the cognitive function of the brain.

2. You can incorporate essential cinnamon into your diet as a blood purifier, which will prevent your face from breaking out in pimples and keep your skin and body feeling fresh.

3. Cinnamon has a therapeutic property that functions as a blood thinner. This blood thinning property aids heart patients, people with high cholesterol, people suffering from pain and people with slow metabolism.

4. For a diabetic patient, cinnamon oil is a good solution to balance blood sugar levels. Reports have suggested that cinnamon oil helps diabetic people control their blood sugar levels.

5. For an arthritic patient, cinnamon oil functions as a pain reliever. It relieves them from muscle and joint pain. Plus, it can reduce the severity of a headache.

6. Cinnamon essential oil is used to accelerate the healing process by stopping the flow of excess blood from cuts and wounds.

7. The oil also eliminates germs found in the gall bladder and bacteria found in staph infections.

8. If you know that heart diseases, high blood pressure problems and high cholesterol are prevalent in your family, then it's vital that you start incorporating cinnamon oil in your meals. In doing so, it will help to decrease your chances of getting these health risks in the future.

9. Another benefit of cinnamon oil is that it reduces your risk of contracting colon cancer.

10. Cinnamon essential oil, a digestive tonic, relieves people suffering from gastric problems. You can use this tonic when suffering from nausea, morning sickness, indigestion, bloating, abdominal cramps, heartburn and vomiting.

11. Take cinnamon essential oil when experiencing symptoms related to sore throat, flu, runny nose and mild congestion.

Applying Cinnamon Essential Oil

1. **Topical Application**- When applying the oil to your skin, combine it with another essential oil, as applying it directly without diluting it first can lead to skin rashes

2. **Aromatic Application**- Cinnamon essential oil-scented candles are a popular purchase among many people. You can light the candles in your home to inhale the smell of cinnamon, put a scented cloth in your car and put them in the bathroom or your room. Furthermore, scented cinnamon oil candles will keep flies from entering your home, as it also functions as a bug repellent.

3. **Internal Application**- Since cinnamon was first used to cook food, it is safe to use cinnamon essential oil when cooking. Therefore, instead of using cinnamon barks, use few drops of cinnamon essential oil to flavor the food.

4. **Sensitive Application**- If you have sensitive skin that is easily irritated, you should dilute the oil and test it on the underside of your arm before applying to the rest of your skin.

Cinnamon Essential Oils: Precautions

a) Cinnamon bark is a very strong type of essential oil. Therefore, it should not be consumed directly.

b) Due to its strong nature, people with acne or other skin diseases should not apply cinnamon essential oil, as applying the oil can aggravate the condition even more.

c) Cinnamon essential should not be applied to any area of the face.

d) You should not inhale the fumes of cinnamon essential oil directly from the bottle or diffuser, instead opt for inhaling it through a cloth, towel or through a candle. Inhaling the fumes directly from the bottle or diffuser can aggravate your nasal passages.

Peppermint Essential Oil

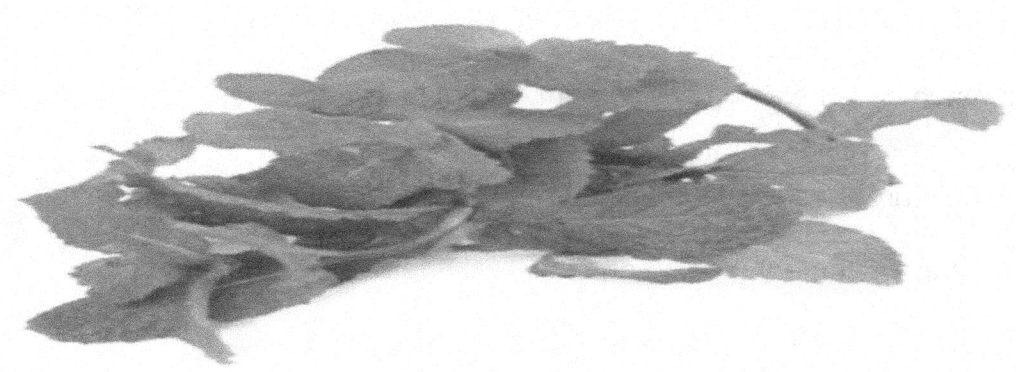

The Healing Powers of Peppermint Essential Oil

When you think of peppermint, you think of candy. However, the word peppermint has a deeper meaning in history.

Way back in ancient times, peppermint was used by the elders to treat problems such as bowel spasms, upset stomach, headaches, fever, respiratory diseases, indigestion and nausea. The wise medical experts of that time recognized the analgesic, antiseptic, antiviral, antibacterial, and anti-inflammatory medical benefits of peppermint. In fact, peppermint is history's oldest and greatest medicine.

Due to its prominent historical status, peppermint is sold in tablet, oil, syrup and capsule form.

The Health Benefits of Peppermint Essential Oil

1. If you have problems digesting your food, often feel bloated and suffer from the agony of constipation, you should start using peppermint essential oil to re-

charge your digestive system. After every major meal, put a few drops of peppermint essential oil into a cold glass of water and drink it. Peppermint essential oil can eliminate the feeling and pain of heartburn as well.

2. People with Irritable Bowel Syndrome (IBS) can relieve the pain and discomfort in the stomach by consuming peppermint essential oil.

3. Many dental care products such as toothpaste or mouthwash are sold with a prominent announcement labeled on their packages stating that they have peppermint in essential oil is extremely useful in treating toothaches.

4. Your nails can also benefit from peppermint essential oil. People prone to getting fungal infections can apply peppermint oil directly to their nails.

5. Headaches and migraines can be prevented with this oil. When you get a headache, dilute the oil and rub it on the temples of your forehead.

6. The next time you feel stressed, anxious or depressed, you should take a long sniff of peppermint oil from a cloth, pillow, or candle. It will help clear your mind.

7. The reason many cough medicines have peppermint in them is because peppermint's strong flavor aids in clearing the respiratory tract. It provides immediate temporary relief from illnesses such as bronchitis, asthma, cold, sinusitis and cough. This led to the development of cold balms and rubs, which are applied to the nasal passages and chest.

8. When in pain, apply cold balms and rubs to your body. It can also be applied to the forehead to reduce fever.

9. People with weak immune systems can use peppermint oil to fend off common diseases. In addition to assisting disease prevention, it also aids in the circulation of blood. In return, the circulation of blood through the entire body boosts metabolism and provides oxygen for the brain. Diabetic, Alzheimer and Dementia patients can benefit from the circulation of blood.

10. Several shampoos are targeted towards people who have an itchy scalp due to lice and dandruff. Shampoos include the ingredient peppermint, which gives off a cooling effect when you put it on your scalp.

11. If you have oily or dull skin, you can use peppermint essential oil to improve the appearance of your skin.

Applying Peppermint Essential Oil

1. **Topical Application** - If you have sensitive skin you will want to diffuse to oil. Other than that, this oil can be applied directly to your skin. However, it's advised to rub small amounts of oil in one area.

2. **Aromatic Application** - You can inhale the smell of the essential oil through a candle or from steam produced when the oil is boiled.

3. **Internal Application** - Peppermint essential oil is safe to use when preparing meals and it can also be taken orally without the need to dilute it.

Peppermint Essential Oil: Precautions

a) Peppermint essential oil should not be put around the eyes, in the ears or inside the nose.

b) Pregnant and nursing women should avoid using peppermint oil.

c) The overuse of peppermint oil can give you headaches, allergic reactions and heartburn.

d) If you want to use peppermint oil for weight loss purposes, then you should ask a doctor first.

Eucalyptus Essential Oil

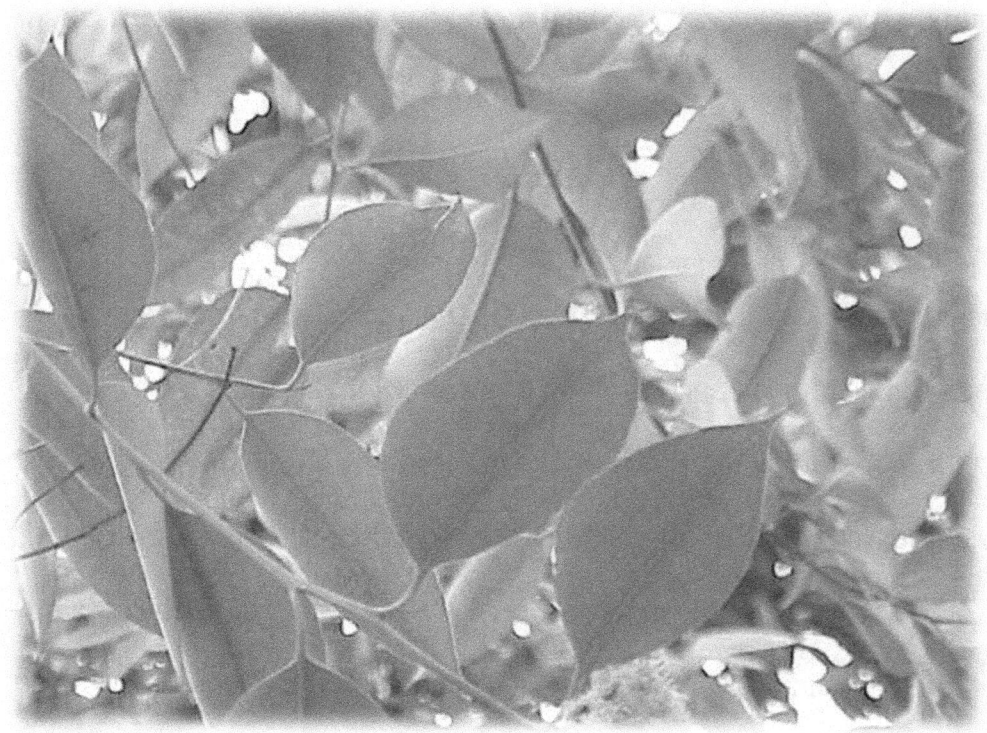

The Healing Powers of Eucalyptus Essential Oil

Eucalyptus essential oil is distilled from the green leaves of the mighty eucalyptus tree.

Only in the past few years, the medical benefits of the eucalyptus became known, and then eucalyptus essential oil was derived from it.

The eucalyptus essential oil's benefits are very similar to the rest of the essential oils. Although it's a fairly new addition to homeopathic practices, eucalyptus oil boasts antiseptic, decongestant, anti-inflammatory and anti-infectious properties.

These medical properties help combat infections and diseases related to the respiratory system, common colds, asthma, and skin damage.

The Health Benefits of Eucalyptus Essential Oil

1. Due to eucalyptus's antiseptic properties, it is used to heal up burns, wounds, abrasions, cuts, sores and ulcers. Eucalyptus oil can be put on fresh and open cuts or wounds to prevent germs or bacteria from entering.

2. Eucalyptus essential oil's expertise lies in treating problems related to the respiratory system. They treat a variety of problems such as cough, flu, sore throat, sinusitis, congestion, and bronchitis. You can combine warm water with some drops of eucalyptus oil and gargle to ease sore throat pain.

3. Asthma can be triggered by fur, dust, smoke, pollen, and humidity. The smallest change in weather can bring on an asthma attack. In order to reduce the occurrence of the attacks, a person needs to take a few drops of eucalyptus oil and rub it on the chest in small round circles. This provides the lungs with oxygen and promotes normal breathing.

4. Mental stress can really dampen one's mood. They feel less energetic and more moody and tired. This lethargic feeling can be prevented by using eucalyptus oil to cool your mind and body, as it works as a stimulant.

5. Eucalyptus oil is a good remedy for people enduring joint pain, stiff muscles, lumbago, sprained ligaments, common body aches, and rheumatism and nerve pain. When putting on eucalyptus oil, move your hands in a circular motion.

6. The oil can also combat cavities, gingivitis and other problems related to dental care. For this reason, eucalyptus oil is found in many dental hygiene products.

7. If you need a natural remedy for treating lice, use eucalyptus oil because it is known as an effective bug repellent. Try not using lice shampoos, as they can

damage your hair. Using eucalyptus oil will not only kill the lice, but will also leave your hair looking shiny and healthily.

8. Sometimes, your intestinal system can contract germs. So, if you fear your intestinal system has bacteria attached to it, you can get rid of them by consuming eucalyptus essential oil by mixing it with another substance.

9. With regular use of eucalyptus oil on your skin, you can say goodbye to skin infections and hello to beautiful and glowing skin.

10. People with diabetes can consume eucalyptus with another substance to control their blood sugar levels. Moreover, diabetes prevents the circulation of blood to occur normally, so ingesting the oil will help the circulation of the blood. Plus, people can even massage oil onto their skin or inhale it to prevent the blood vessels from constricting.

11. Eucalyptus oil is also widely recognized as "fever oil." The nickname refers to their ability to reduce the fever.

12. Symptoms of tuberculosis and pneumonia are very painful. Rubbing eucalyptus oil on your back and chest can help to reduce the symptoms associated with tuberculosis and pneumonia.

ApplyingEucalyptus Essential Oil

1. **Topical Application**- You can apply eucalyptus directly to your skin, without diluting it.

2. **Aromatic Application**- Eucalyptus oil is often used as a room freshener at hospitals to keep the air clean. You can spray it around your house to kill the germs and bacteria.

3. **Internal Application**- Before you ingest it, be sure to dilute it first.

4. **Sensitive Application**- You can find out if eucalyptus oil irritates your skin or not by applying a small amount of oil on your skin.

Eucalyptus Essential Oil: Precautions

a) Since research on eucalyptus oil is scarce, it's recommended that you consume it in small amounts instead of large.

b) Taking more than three drops of eucalyptus oil can lead to many complications. The side effects of taking large quantities of undiluted oil can result in stomach cramps, burning, muscle weakness, nausea, vomiting, and dizziness.

c) It's safe for pregnant and breastfeeding women to use eucalyptus oil.

d) At least two weeks prior to going under the knife, you should stop taking eucalyptus oil as it lowers the blood sugar levels.

Chamomile Essential Oil

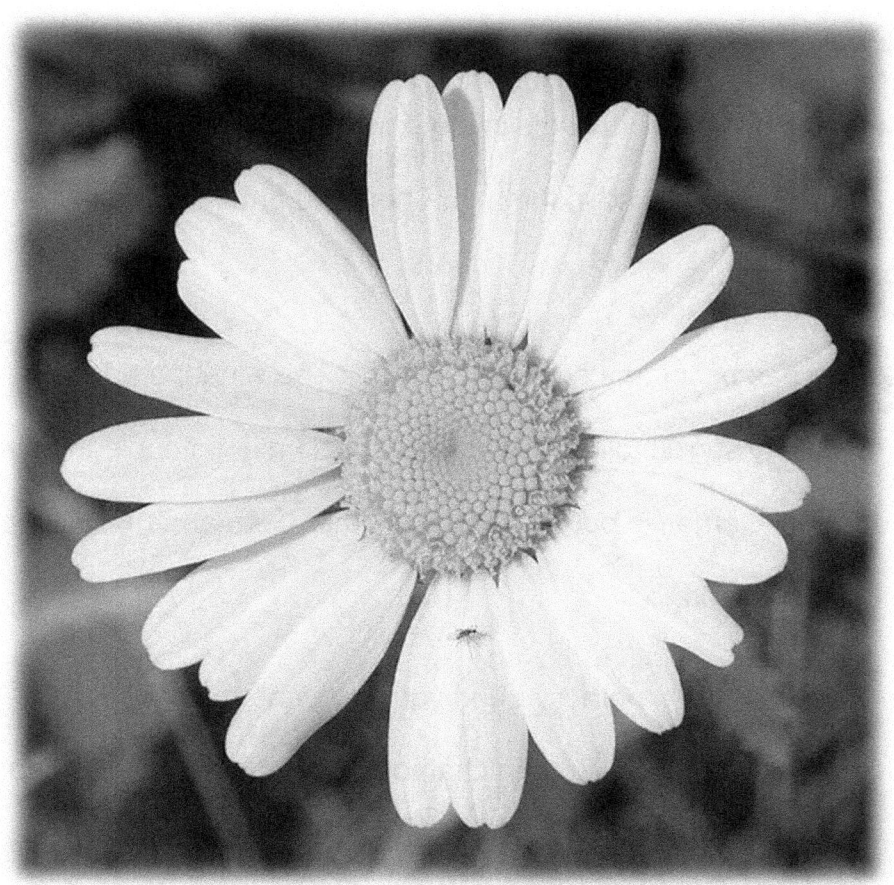

Healing Powers of Chamomile Essential Oil

There are two types of chamomile plants. One is called the Roman chamomile plant

and the other is called the German chamomile plant. These two types of plants,

although different in names, have similar medicinal benefits. They both have anti-

inflammatory, calming, anti-parasitic, anti-infectious, and relaxing medical properties.

The both are capable of treating such illnesses as indigestion, frostbite, eczema, sore

throat, wounds, sore gums, liver problems, sinusitis and gallbladder problems, diaper

rash in infants and other conditions. Although most of the medical benefits they provide are similar, there are a few differences between the two that will be individually addressed.

The Health Benefits of Chamomile Essential Oil

1. German and Roman essential oil both can eliminate worms from the intestines. They can also kill lice and mites found in the hair. They also protect your hair and scalp from contracting infections.

2. These days depression has become a common disease. The widespread lethargy, stress and anxiety surrounding people has caused many people to rely on prescription drugs. An alternative option is to take either German or Roman essential oil to battle depression.

3. Do you have small kids who are hyperactive and you just want them to calm down? If you do, then you should use Roman chamomile oil to assist them to pay more attention to other important things, like their schoolwork.

4. The German chamomile oil contains medicinal properties that help treat inflammation located in the urinary or digestive system of adults. This oil will also help to lower your blood pressure.

5. Both these oils assist the functioning of the abdomen tract by regulating the digestive system's secretion process to enable digestion. More importantly, the oils assist the bile in exiting from the liver properly.

6. The German and Roman chamomile essential oil restarts the circulatory system into functioning efficiently, and then it removes toxins from the blood. The

restarting and removal process helps to treat arthritis and rheumatism. Also, it decreases edema and swelling.

7. Girls around the world should rejoice, as both the German and Roman chamomile essential oil help decrease the appearance of scars and dark spots on the face and skin. So, if you have scars due acne or pimples, use these oils to diminish them.

8. These chamomile essential oils work as a disinfectant as well. If you happen to get cuts, bruises or wounds, rub this oil on top of them to create a shield of protection from germs in the air.

9. In case of high fever, use Roman or German chamomile essential oil. Using either one these oils will make you sweat, thus reducing the fever, and removing toxins from your body.

10. Another benefit both these oils have is that they work well in decreasing muscle and joint pain. Furthermore, use these oils when you have a headache, injuries bone, toothache, or congestion.

11. Both types of oil work as a gas eliminator, meaning they expel gas out of the body and stop it from forming in the stomach.

12. German and Roman chamomile essential oil will keep your nervous system in check by reducing spasms and convulsions.

Applying Chamomile Essential Oil

1. **Topical Application**- Roman and German chamomile can be applied to skin. If you wish you could dilute it with another essential oil, but it is safe to put on the skin directly.

2. **Aromatic Application**- You can put the Roman or German essential oil in bathtubs while bathing. This is a good method to inhale the smell of the oils. People suffering from hay fever, sore throat, sinus inflammation and ear inflammation can inhale the fumes.

3. **Internal Application**- Roman and German chamomile is often mixed in food and drinks to give them flavor. People can also ingest these essential oils by combining them with other oils to cure infections in the liver and gallbladder.

4. **Sensitive Application**- If you do not have sensitive skin, then you can directly apply to the skin without testing it on your arm. However, it's advised that before you put any type of oil on your arm, you should test it first.

Chamomile Essential Oils: Precautions

a) Roman and German chamomile has been deemed safe to consume, but if taken in large quantities, it can cause vomiting.

b) If you are allergic to chamomile, then you should try another essential oil and avoid using oils containing chamomile.

c) Avoid using Roman and German chamomile oil during pregnancy and when nursing because they have been reported to have caused miscarriages.

Tea Tree Essential Oil

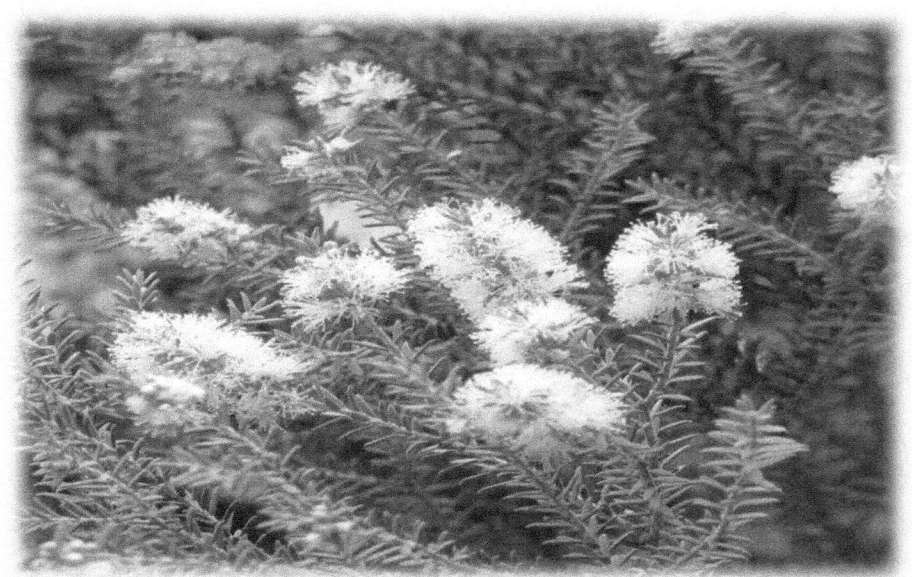

Healing Powers of Tea Tree Essential Oil

Tea tree oil, not to be mistaken for tea oil, is oil that's extracted from trees found in Australia. In Australia, it is a "go-to" medicine for treating wounds, cuts, bruises and other ailments. Tea tree essential oil is made up of antioxidant, antiviral, digestive, antifungal, antiseptic and other medicinal properties.

The numerous amounts of properties tea tree oil contain makes it an unbeatable force to treat diseases and illnesses.

The Health Benefits of Tea Tree Essential Oil

1. Tea Tree oil can be taken to treat and cure dangerous and life-threatening wounds infected by bacteria. Therefore, applying this oil as soon as possible to your wound can help prevent the occurrence of bacterial infections. Moreover, it can also treat infections in the stomach, colon, intestines and urinary system and excretory system.

2. If you ever contract malaria or hay fever, then tea tree essential oil can eliminate the bacteria causing you to become ill.

3. Have you noticed that each year you have either the flu or a cold? The reason for this is that common illnesses always find a way to fool the immune system. The common illnesses change and adapt to your body. In order to damage them, you can use tea tree oil. Tea tree oil will treat all kinds of viral infections that include curing mumps, pox, flu and measles.

4. Tea tree essential oil helps your body absorb nutrients from food, which in return protects your body from diseases.

5. As discussed above, tea tree oil is mostly used to treat wounds and protect them from infections.

6. For the skin, you can use tea tree oil to reduce scars caused by boils, acne, eruptions and pimples.

7. Tea tree oil can treat bronchitis, congestion, cold and cough. While sleeping, rub some tea tree oil on your chest or put it on your pillow to inhale its scent overnight.

8. You can use the oil to treat athlete's foot and for other bacterial and fungal infections. If you happen to get an internal fungal disease, it's advised that you don't ingest tea tree oil, as it is highly toxic. However, you can try other herbal remedies.

9. If you need a quick fix to solving your dandruff problems and hair loss problems, massage your head with tea tree oil. It will make your hair shine, and at the same time get rid of hair-related problems.

10. Tea tree oil strengthens your immune system and shields you from contracting infections. It also helps to regulate the flow of blood. Since you can't consume it, you can stick to inhaling the odors produced by the tea tree oil.

Applying Tea Tree Essential Oil

Topical Application-Since tea tree essential oil's main use is to be applied on open cuts or wounds, it's safe to say that you can apply it on to your skin.

Aromatic Application- You can apply tea tree oil on pillowcases, clothes or even buy candles emanating the aroma of the oils.

Internal Application- Tea tree essential oil should never be taken orally—doing so can be lethal.

Tea Tree Essential Oil: Precautions

a) Tea tree oil if taken orally can cause a rash, a coma, hallucinations, inability to

walk, dizziness, upset stomach, rashes and confusion.

b) Tea tree oil under no circumstances should be given to pets and children.

Is it Safe to Use Essential Oils?

Each type of essential oil comes with its own set of warnings. In order to be safe, you should follow the following guidelines to gain a better understanding of using essential oils safely.

General Guidelines of Using Essential Oils

Following are some rules you should follow, before you start using essential oils:

1. There are some essential oils that can be hazardous if applied directly to your skin. These oils can cause your skin to burn. So always remember to dilute them first with another essential oil or combine it with water. By combining two oils or oil with water together, the toxicity levels of the oils will lower. Therefore, if an essential oil has high toxicity levels, you will need to combine it with an essential oil that has low toxicity levels.

2. Never let essential oils stay on your skin for too long, as they can lead to rashes.

3. Essential oils, even if pure, can be toxic for your body. Therefore, you should always read the label to determine the toxicity levels of essential oils.

4. Avoid putting essential oils in body openings such as the ears, mouth and nose.

5. Overdosing on essential oils can cause you to have immense headaches and severe dizziness. So, if you happen to use essential oils to make a candle or soap, remember to do it in an open area.

6. If you have small children or pets in the house, put your oils in a place they cannot reach and, as an extra precaution, remember to lock the cupboard as well.

7. Essential oils are highly combustible. So keep lighters, matches and other flammable devices or sources separate from essential oils.

8. Prior to using essential oils, you should consult your doctor. If you have a preexisting medical condition, then it's advised to consult your doctor first.

What to Do In Case Of Emergencies

If an allergic reaction occurs or if someone swallows essential oils by accident, then these are the following measure you need take:

1. If the essential oil gets into your eyes, ears or any other body openings by accident, you should immediately take a cold glass of milk and rinse your face with it. After few hours, if the condition worsens, you should see a doctor.

2. If essential oils get on your hands, rinse your hands with mild soap. However, if the oil remains stuck on your hands, you can use vegetable or coconut oil to get it off your hands.

3. If you or someone you know swallows an essential oil that is not to be consumed, immediately take them to the nearest hospital.

4. If a pet happens to consume it, take them to a veterinarian.

Patch Testing Method

You should first choose the type of oil you want to use, and then dilute it with filtered water. Combine at least three to four drops with the filtered water. Then go ahead and put it on your elbow or the underside of your arm or legs. Then proceed to cover the area with a bandage, but remember not to get this area wet. After 24 hours, you can remove the bandage to find out if you are allergic to that oil or not.

The patch testing method is pertinent when using essential oils, as it determines if you are allergic to them or not.

Conclusion

Nature has brought you essential oils for healing, and to aid in using therapeutic methods to prevent diseases and illnesses. There are over 100 essential oils that nature has gifted you. Instead of relying solely on modern medicine, it is worth also trying essential healing oils. If they worked for your ancestors, then they can work for you as well. It's time that you fully embrace what nature has provided you with.

Nature has given you its miracle so you can explore its benefits. So, go on and take your pick from the numerous lists of essential oils to find out which one suits your needs.